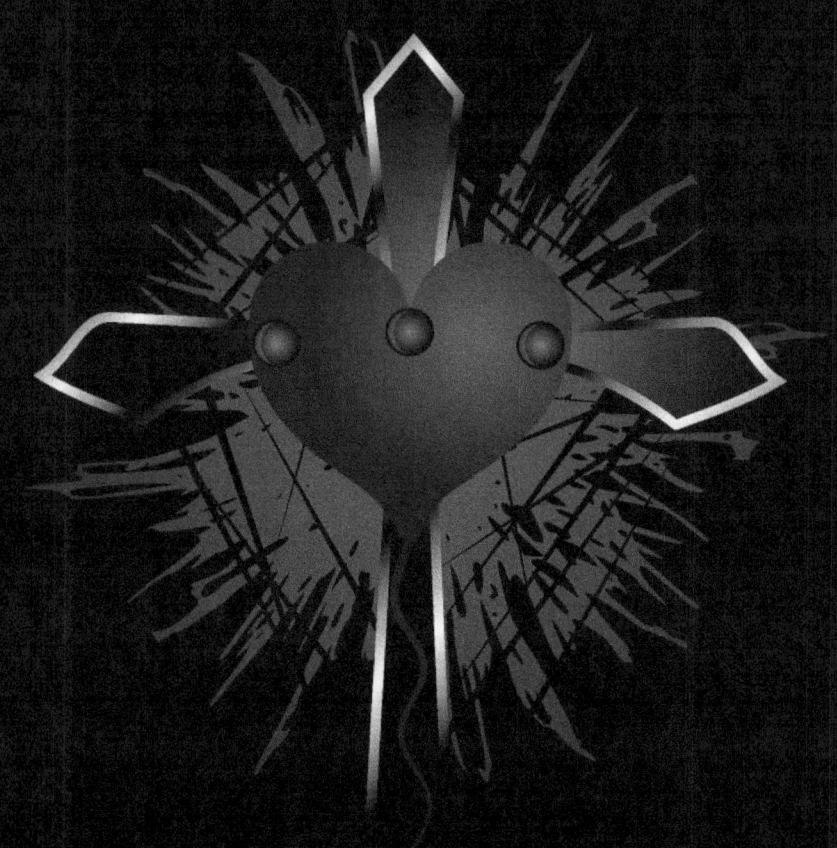

When Pain Gives You Hope COVID-19

By Sederia Graves

Cover Created by Jazzy Kitty Publications

Logo Designs by Andre M. Saunders/Jess Zimmerman

Editor: Anelda L. Attaway

Co-editor: Sederia G. Graves

© 2021 Sederia Graves

ISBN 978-1-954425-22-4

Library of Congress Control Number: 2021905345

All rights reserved. This book is protected by the copyright laws of the United States of America. This book may not be copied or reprinted for commercial gain or profit. The use of short quotations or occasional page copying for personal or group study is permitted and encouraged. Permission will be granted upon request. For Worldwide Distribution. Printed in the United States of America. Published by Jazzy Kitty Publishing utilizing Microsoft Publishing Software and Book Coverly. The Holy Scriptures are from the Holy Bible.

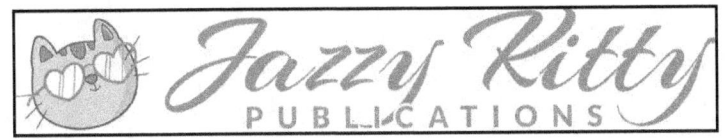

ACKNOWLEDGMENTS

First and foremost, the Most High God and my steadfast belief in the Word of God. Thank You for choosing me for this miracle; I am humbled and blessed forever.

Thank my family, My siblings, Michael, Eva, and Pattie, for your support and prayers.

Thank you to my Sons, Michael, Jason, and Bryson Adolphus, for the love and support you both gave to your sister and for keeping the faith along with her for my recovery.

My Nieces, Alisha and Shekinah.

My best friend Pam and favorite cousin Dominique.

Thank my church and Pastors Cory Condrey and Joann Rosario Condrey at Rainfire Church in Douglasville, GA.

Thank the doctors and nurses who took care of me and never gave up on my care.

Last but not least, every person who prayed for me and all of those who donated to my Go Fund Me Page, it was the blessing I needed to keep me going once I came home.

DEDICATIONS

This book is dedicated to my beautiful Daughter Airedes Theresa Bruce. I know that this experience changed your whole life, but I never heard anything but good from every person I talked to after coming home from the hospital.

Thank you for keeping everyone informed, for taking care of your younger brother in my absence through this difficult time.

Thank you for standing strong in your faith and having a warrior spirit that would not give up no matter what the doctors told you.

Thanks for believing for me when I could not believe for myself; blessings to you forever.

Love your Mom

TABLE OF CONTENTS

INTRODUCTION	i
STAGE 1	01
STAGE 2	05
STAGE 3	26
STAGE 4	31
STAGE 5	38
STAGE 6	44
STAGE 7	50
ABOUT THE AUTHOR	54

INTRODUCTION

As you read this publication, many of you, like myself, won't realize the purpose or value and why I take pictures of me, my children, and grandchildren. It is because I almost died a year ago, at least the old me did because of a severe COVID-19 experience.

It dawned on me after Father God was so gracious to spare my life how little value I gave to living and the lives of my family members. So, I am not taking pictures out of vanity but gratitude for how miraculously God has healed me (spiritually, emotionally, and physically). I was spared to see my 2nd grandchild's birth, Prince Marcus Joshua. My 30-year-old (Nobleman Bryson Adolphus) made it through horrendous drug addiction and is getting sober today. My daughter, a soldier for righteousness and faith Airedes (the Goddess), became and still is that soldier for Father God. God bridged the gap between me and my oldest son King Michael Jason (one who is like God), after 18 years of distancing. My true best friends are still my best friends today. I came to realize through this experience how much my siblings love me. Lastly, how many lives I've touched without knowing through ministering God's Word with a wonderful Man of God. I could go on.

God is amazing in what He blessed me to experience and through what was viewed as the worst but yet, the most miraculous life-changing event. This publication shares a small piece of how I became "Pastor Amazing Grace," and I am beyond grateful.

Pastor A. G. Graves

STAGE 1

Wow, I never thought I would get COVID-19 because I did everything right. I remember the night, well actually, it was early morning; I was up coloring my picture "Rebirth." It was raining heavily with much thunder and lightning, and all of a sudden, I heard this really loud clap of thunder. It was so tremendous that the whole house literally shook. I knew then something had entered the earth realm that was powerful and evil. The thought came to my mind immediately, as stated in Revelations 12:10, about the adversary being thrown from Heaven to earth like a bolt of lightning. And if any of you know about the weather, lightning comes first and then the thunder.

It was in October 2019 when I heard this thunder. I knew in my heart of hearts (my spirit man) that something had entered our atmosphere that we were not aware of and that it was something we needed to get prepared for by praying and seeking God for answers. I don't remember timewise how long after this occurrence that the Spirit of God spoke to me and told me to prepare my house. It was the same anointing the doorpost as the children of Israel did in the old testament when they wanted the death angel to pass over their homes (which is where Passover comes from). God was sending a decree (plague) among the people for the sake of delivering His people from bondage, and all of the first-born males of every household would die. He specifically let me know in my spirit man to anoint my children, myself, and the doorpost of my home. He also told me to pray and stand to intercede for other family members who were not present in my home.

I did as the Spirit instructed me to do, and I anointed and prayed with my children. I made a couple of calls to a few people who were on my heart and told them the same thing. I remember the last time something similar to this happened when I lived in California, and the Spirit of God spoke to me and told me the same thing but with specifics about the death angel coming into the earth realm. I witnessed so many deaths in a short period of time all over the country, from people I knew to people who were well known all over the world in entertainment, sports, etc., old and young. I learned from that experience when the Spirit of the Lord speaks to me in this manner to be obedient, and then I am.

"Now, some of you may not be believers in the Most High God or Jesus Christ, but I am an advocate for Christ and I need to make this proclamation clear before telling the rest of this story. It will be key; I believe in exalting the power and authenticity of the God that I serve. I believe Him to be the one and true Living God."

I didn't question God as to why I needed to do this; I just moved in obedience to the intensity of this, knowing in my being I needed to follow the instruction that was clear to me in my heart. The first thing that occurred was that somewhere between December 2018 and October 2019, My son and I had experienced a severe cough prior to the announcing of COVID that lasted for an unusual period of time. Even with that, going to the doctor seemed useless because I remember specifically my Primary Care Physician saying this severe cough had been going around, and they were not quite sure what it was. But they were treating it as if it was a virus and using antibiotics along with another pill that was supposed to dryup the mucus in the chest and congestion.

I believe COVID-19 had already entered our mist, but the medical profession didn't know what it was. In the meantime, it evolved into the second strand of COVID, which began to rear its ugly head coming into the beginning of 2020. People were getting this thing, but because the doctors were not familiar with it, they misdiagnosed and treated it incorrectly because they didn't even know what it was or that it existed. As this evil disease (strand) mutated, the illness and its effects worsened and became a threat to our society. They put a name to it and realized whatever it was, they didn't know how to treat it, and the reaction from the disease was becoming more rapid and deadly.

I recall going to the doctor and being treated for that persistent cough twice, but it held on to me for about four months and my son for about six months. It was horrible and created severe chest pains and soreness. The cough was dry and so difficult that your stomach muscles were sore, and it would sometimes even cause vomiting, but they didn't know what it was, so they treated it as though it was a virus. Finally, after suffering from that for about 4 to 6 months, my son and I began to get well, and it just went away. I thought, okay, we are over this thing, whatever it was, this happened before the thunder and lightning incident.

Sometimes we can take our faith foolishly because we think one thing when God intends for us to use wisdom in all things. When the government began to shut down the states, although I believed the virus was real, I didn't take the precautions that I should have by using a mask, gloves and sanitizing my hands. I just thought because God had already prepared me for the coming of this ugly virus, I was protected. I was in the process of moving, and so many other things were happening in my lifethat I was trying to figure out. My focus was not on using wisdom and following the regulations and rules to help keep us well and safe from spreading or catching this virus.

I was out and about without a mask and just trying to move from one place to another so that I would be settled in somewhere. Then I could take the COVID thing a little more seriously once I finished what I needed to do. I knew God would protect me because I had anointed my doorpost and my family, so I wasn't worried about it at all. Little did I know that I would fall victim to this horrible disease myself to a degree that I could have never imagined.

STAGE 2

After we got moved into our new place, and I didn't remember this until after I had been through the whole COVID-19 experience; I never anointed my new home. Although I prayed for doors to be opened to get the new home, I didn't cover it in prayer as I had the home that I moved from because that's where I was living when that storm came, and the Spirit of God originally spoke to me. I am sure at some point, I was reminded in my spirit to anoint the house I had moved into, but I didn't do it. I want to bring these points out because I want to enlighten us to be more aware of the nudging in our spirits when our Creator strives to make us aware of things to come. We get so busy doing us that we forget that we're only able to do that because the Creator of all things gives us continuous life and breath daily.

We have edged God out of our lives so much with technology and all of these things that He has given us the mind to create. We forget that the Creator is still the reason for every living, moving, and breathing thing that we see around us every day. We forget that all of the luxuries that we have been gifted to create and enjoy start from something that was already created that had nothing to do with humanity. The raw materials, oceans, stars, moon, sun, clouds so many things around us that are out of our control are the very things we utilize to make many of the things that we use day to day. Our Creator created us in His image and likeness so that we could also be creators, but we will never be able to create certain things or fully explain their existence no matter how hard we strive to understand.

We moved into our new home on March 21st, and the state was already on curfew and may have been shut down. My recollection of that is not the greatest, or I believe the state was shut down shortly thereafter. I remember running errands to get everything in place for the new house, having people come for the cable, installing the washer and dryer, and many other things you do when you first move. Many people have asked me if I knew who I got it from, and I can only tell you it is an invisible disease because you can have it and not know that you have it, so to answer that question, no, I had no idea. I was out and about a lot after we moved, going here and there. I was eating on the run and putting things in storage. The only thing that did stand out in my mind is I remember thinking that I had really been struggling with my asthma more than usual, it seemed.

About a week after we moved in, I went to the doctor to check on my asthma. By this time, the state was already shut down because they were not doing too many face-to-face appointments. I did actually go in to see a doctor, but he was very hesitant about being in the room with me. He came in fully covered and barely touched me. I told him my symptoms, and I don't even recall him listening to my chest or anything. However, he prescribed me a breathing machine and albuterol medicine to go into the machine. He advised me to take a treatment every night and whenever I felt like it was really difficult for me to breathe. I took the machine, went home, and just followed his instructions. But it didn't seem like it was getting better nor seem to be getting worse. Looking back on it now, I am pretty sure with what is now known about COVID; I had it at that first doctor's visit. Had a chest X-ray been taken, they would have caught it sooner. All things considered, the medical profession at that time was as ignorant about the disease as the public.

I was taking the treatments regularly at this point which was unusual because I never had to use a breathing machine before in the life of my asthma. Nevertheless, since I am getting older, I just took it as it was pollen season, and I had just moved; I assumed I was just struggling a little more than usual. This was before they started telling you what signs to look out for, with shortness of breath being one of them. I took the treatments regularly for about 2 (two) weeks. In the meantime, we were still unpacking boxes and striving to figure out how we would fit everything in the house since we were downsizing. I remember a couple of days before I went to the urgent care on or about April 19th, I had finally emptied all of the boxes in the house except for one, and I managed to push it into my closet.

I went into the living room where my daughter was sitting and said to her, "Wow, I finally got all of the boxes emptied except one, but I feel really tired."

She said to me, "Well, Mom, you gotta remember you are not as young as you used to be. It is probably from all of the moving and working you have been doing to get everything in order. Why don't you just rest."

Taking into consideration what she said, I thought that is exactly what I will do. I vaguely remember what happened next, so some of the dialogue you hear from this point will be shared information from what I can remember and what was told to me from my daughter. She became the advocate for all of the decision-making about my care from when I went into the hospital until I came home.

Little did I know that this night would start a journey through illness that I had never experienced before and hoped to never experience again in my lifetime. I remember getting in the bed and then feeling like I couldn't breathe well, so I got up to take a breathing treatment with the breathing machine I had used several nights in a row, still thinking I was having a hard time with my asthma. I also remember that night being in pain in my back and feeling that I might have a fever. I understand that a good friend of mine came over to bring some natural products for congestion and sorts and rub me down with Tiger balm. I felt like I might be coming down with something, but still, I didn't feel like I was sick enough to go to the hospital.

My friend told my daughter and me that if I didn't seem to be better, he suggested that I go to the hospital. I was hesitant because, with the rules set in place about the virus, I just didn't want to be separated from my family nor be quarantined or isolated. I went to sleep and this part of the story is what was told to me by my daughter because my memory of this is extremely vague and on and off. My daughter said she spoke to me the following morning as always, but she noticed that I was lying at the foot of my bed horizontally and not in the bed under the covers like usual. She spoke and went into the office (which is at the other end of our house from the bedroom). She stated that although she was working, she was just bothered in her spirit about me, and she just kept being nudged to come and see if I was okay.

She came back into my room right around 11 a.m. and questioned me again about how I was doing, and I let her know I wasn't feeling too well, but she also noticed that I was barely breathing, or at least it appeared that way to her. She said she roused me and told me she was going to take me to the hospital because I wasn't breathing right. I stated I didn't want to go because they would keep me, and I didn't want to be separated from her and her brother. I can say today I am glad she was so persistent. She packed me up and took me over to the Kaiser facility in Kennesaw, GA.; It was their urgent care facility. I don't remember most of the ride to the urgent care, but I do remember just as we pulled up and her getting the wheelchair so I could be pushed into the facility rather than me trying to walk. Once she got me to the entrance, they told her she would not be able to come into the facility with me and just to wait to find out what the final diagnosis would be once they ran some tests.

I am sure they did the usual things such as temperature check and blood pressure. I don't remember what was said or what orders were requested, but there had to be a chest X-ray because I still have the copy of the X-ray on my phone. Once there, it was established that I had double pneumonia and that my lungs, as stated, were very sick. It was also diagnosed that I was only breathing at 10% of oxygen, meaning that they had to give me 90% of oxygen. I was literally almost dead. The point I want to bring out is that I didn't even know that I was that sick. I didn't feel that sick; I was just unpacking boxes and running errands as usual and just feeling a little tired. If I had not gone to the hospital, there would have been no way, based on how I felt, that you could have convinced me that I was really that sick and barely breathing on my own. I don't remember breathing heavy, gasping for air, or coughing.

Once it was established that I wasn't going back home, the communication regarding my care would be over the phone or FaceTime from this point. I still am not completely sure as to whether it was the next day or the day after, a conference call was made to my daughter. Who, in turn, included her brothers on the call about my condition and that even though they had been giving me oxygen, the breathing seemed as though it had not changed. My condition was not improving; therefore, they needed to make some changes and adjustments to keep me around and preserve my life. They needed to do something that would help improve my breathing and something that could take the pressure off of my lungs, and at this point, my heart was overworking. They talked to my daughter about putting me in an induced coma. I was against it because someone very dear to us passed away after being placed in an induced coma, and we lost him in the process, so a part of it was fear, and the other part was just not knowing if it was going to work. At this point, and having been given the diagnosis that I did have COVID, my daughter was forced to decide that would or could determine my life and my death. As she explained to me, to do nothing was not an option, so with my participation and family members, we chose to allow them to put me in an induced coma with the understanding that I would be awakened every day. I am not sure in what order or how many days apart these things happened. I do know it all happened in a matter of days and in the switching of hospitals. I originally went to Kaiser Urgent Care and from there, I was transferred to St. Joseph's Emory Hospital in Dunwoody, GA. Emory is thought to be one of the best hospital care facilities in GA, so I was in good hands medically, but as my story continues, you will find that I was in the best hands ever spiritually.

The initial concern was getting my breathing or oxygen levels up from the 10% breathing number, and yet even though the decision was made to place me on a ventilator, my breathing only improved by 10%. Now I was still having to receive oxygen at 80%. This was a concern for the physicians because the necessity of me being put to sleep was in hopes that it would assist in helping my lungs to begin to get well so that my breathing capacity would increase but still to no avail. The next step was striving to find out what was blocking my breathing, so in order for them to open up an airway, they needed to put a breathing tube in my chest. I can only assume that another x-ray of the chest was taken because the next decision was to open up the lung that had now collapsed, which contributed to the breathing problem. I later learned from one of my sons that a bubble was discovered as part or all of the blockage between my lung being revitalized and my breathing improving drastically. So, they needed to place the tube in to dissipate the bubble.

In the process of actually striving to get me well, it seemed as though my body was working against me because of the rapid effect of COVID in the body. The attack is so swift that the timing of each thing they did was imperative to my ability to get well. Once the breathing apparatus was in place, tube in the chest, ventilator, and a tracheotomy in the throat, they slowly began to see an increase in my oxygen levels. But now they had a problem with my heart pumping blood through my organs the way it needed to for my survival and the preservation of my other organs. The next decision that had to be made was what is referred to as ECMO, which is generally a form of life support. They had to place a tube in my heart to pump the blood in and out of my heart outside of my body so it could be purified as well as pumped in and out for proper circulation to sustain my organs.

Here I am in a coma, ECMO life support, tracheotomy, a tube in my throat intubated, and a ventilator breathing for me. My son told me that they were allowed to talk with me every day while I was comatose, and they would have FaceTime and just talk to me. My three children, my siblings, and other closest relatives. They would also pray for me regularly, sing to me, read, etc. All things considered, my body was shutting down as they were striving to revive it and bring life back into my body and organs before they shut down completely. At this point, I was living because of all of the machinery they had placed in or outside of my body doing the work for me that because I was so ill, my body couldn't do on its own. I like you in hearing all of what happened to me outside of my body just became teary-eyed at the miraculous work of God to save me and bring me back to a place of functioning normally and on my own.

In my mind, my experience was very scary. I knew something was happening to me, but I felt totally helpless. I remember having these delusional dreams. I will strive to explain each awakening as it seemed as though I was in a submarine and everyone who was attending to me was of a foreign ethnicity. They were either Asian or Jamaican or African by the dialect I heard. It seemed like the people were far away even though they were in the same room as I was. I knew they were in the room because, in my mind's eye, I could see them, and they didn't look like real people. They looked like plastic manikins. I could hear them speaking to me, but I couldn't answer them out loud, but I could understand them because they were not speaking a foreign language.

The next thing that must have been delusional that began to happen that I believed was really happening is I thought I was being used to create some type of program that required the use of my limbs to make everything look real to whomever this television programming was being shown to. I understood it to be children and that I was hooked up to these electrodes that once transmitted to the room or television screen that they were transmitting to, would look like a butterfly or an animation of some sort. As I moved and/or spoke, those who were watching would see the animation content but not me, nor would they be aware that I existed on the other side of what they were watching. This went on for some period of time and was a regular daily routine. I knew that each day they would come and clean me and prepare me for this "work" of sorts, and somehow, I had the understanding that this was a way of paying for my hospital stay or working it off. This was as real as me telling this story. It wasn't foggy at all. These were clear pictures that I could see in the room where I was staying. They would ask me each day if I was ready to do this work and they would tell me, today you are going to be a butterfly or a flower. All I understood was that whoever could see me was on the other side of the wall and to them, I would appear to be like an electric light show.

Being in the room alone and being incapacitated to help myself in any way was the most stressful part of being in the hospital and being in ICU. As I began to have more conscious hours, I had more delusional stages that I went through that seemed very real. I was in a lot of pain, but it was more of a spiritual distress that medicine could not soothe. There were all kinds of machines that I was attached to. One of the things that were done constantly was the clearing of the sputum from my mouth as I coughed profusely regularly. There was this pump that they would use to suck up the mucus and sputum, and when they used it, I would cough as if I was choking. I assume the coughing was necessary, seeing that I had double pneumonia and needed to release as much of the infection from my lungs as possible. Still, it was so painful and frightening when I began the coughing because sometimes it seemed as though I wasn't going to stop, and I couldn't catch my breath. This went on every day and all the time. My thirst was so bad because I couldn't drink water with the ECMO and the chest and throat restrictions.

I remember a conversation about a mouse getting into the line of the tube that led to my throat, which is when the coughing started. It seemed as though I could see something that appeared to be a mouse in the lines that lead to my respirator/ventilator. The staff spoke about it in a whispering tone to not alarm me, but it left me feeling anxious.

The next dream was about being stuck in a house that was on fire but was also rat-infested in the basement of the home and how we were trying to get rid of the rats through flooding. I had this dream repeatedly and whenever I would awaken from this dream, I would look in the medication line. I wanted to make sure that what appeared to be a mouse was still in the ceiling that led to the ventilator, which led to my tracheotomy tube. I remember the taste and smell of dog hair in my taste buds and in my nose. I had the constant smell of dog hair and tickling in my throat as if I had a blockage preventing me from coughing up this mucus stuck in my throat. The frustration of not letting people know what I was thinking or how I felt was so utterly frightening more than anything else. I couldn't talk, so I attempted to get them to understand that I wanted to write something down. I don't know if it was the medication or the fact that my muscles just weren't strong enough, but I couldn't even write. I couldn't bring my thoughts together to spell or remember certain words to describe what I could clearly hear in my head. It was like my brain had disconnected itself from my body and all of its functions.

I think one of the worst things was not having someone that you know who has your best interest at heart as an advocate for you. Not knowing the people who are caring for you. Some of the staff were very gentle and some of the staff were just doing a job, and they treated you as such they didn't have the patience or caring attitude that in the stages of sickness I was in was needed as a way of knowing that I would be okay. On so many days, I was there just wondering, and I still did not fully understand even why I was there. The assumption was that I remembered how I got there or why I was there, and I didn't. Waking up to an overwhelming amount of machinery and not remembering why you were even there was so scary. I remember going through the thoughts in my mind that maybe I had a fatal car accident and perhaps I killed someone. Maybe I blacked out or fell asleep and really hurt someone, and I was the surviving person. I would hear the staff talking about someone dying and hearing my sister's name being spoken more than once. Eva Brown and saying that she was deceased, yet later once I was made aware of why I was there, and things began to normalize, I realized that I hadn't hurt anyone, nor was my sister deceased. Just lying there, not knowing, would bring tears to my eyes, and I would cry but couldn't even tell anyone why I was crying.

My anxiety and fear were so high that they began to give me anxiety medicine along with all the other medicines they were administering. They would make like the frozen yogurt drink that consisted of all of the meds that I needed to take in pill form as well as the medicines that I had to take intravenously. They would crush them all up and put them in a large syringe and feed it into one of the tubes designated for that and then flush it out once it was administered. It made me think of frozen yogurt, and I knew when they did this, I would get some relief from my pain. The pain was horrible. It was so bad that I couldn't even put words to it. I hurt everywhere, from my head to my toes, literally. My hair even hurt because of my fever. My scalp was tender, and just as I am writing this in no particular order, that is how my brain was working in no particular order. My thoughts were everywhere, so many questions in my mind. I had so many emotions going on at one time. I felt so out of order, like I couldn't pull my thoughts together to make sense of any of what I was experiencing or hearing. Wondering why or how I could be that sick and could not see any of my relatives.

Okay, so let me go back to the dreams and visions that I had while I was there. After going through this process every morning, this seemed to be processed every day to be used for this job of using my body to create some kind of electrical animation. Then they would go through the process of moving me and changing my position. Supposedly to keep me from getting bed sores and breakdowns in my skin. I am really trying to create a picture for you as to what this experience was like because it was really very dark spiritually, a very dark place to see and experience. It was frightening, lonely, cold, and uncaring; it was a feeling of loneliness that there are not words enough to describe. I never felt so helpless and hopeless in my life, and I have had many experiences devastating enough for me to quit, but this was a fight I just couldn't win without some divine intervention and I knew in my heart I couldn't win.

The next thing that I would dream about was being a rat in a maze. I knew that the rat symbolizes me. I could hear over and over there is only one way out and you have to find your way. While going through the maze, I would encounter all kinds of elicit extremes and behaviors while trying to find my way out. The women that I kept coming in contact with seem to be witches who were trying to block me from getting out of the maze. Each time I would go through the maze and come to a dead-end it felt as though I would have a seizure. It would be this intense tightening of every part of my body as if an electrical current were being put through my body like what I imagine electrocution would feel like. It was horrible and painful, and I would wake up in sweat and tears and not want to be put back to sleep, but I knew once I was given my meds, I was going to fall asleep whether I wanted to go to sleep or not. As soon as I was asleep or consciously unaware, this same exact dream would start all over again, and each time I would get to the place in the maze where I was at a dead-end. I could hear a voice saying, *"Sederia, there is only one way out and you have to find it."* Every different dream or experience in the spiritual realm was so dark, but it was all related to the COVID experience. In spite of the different experiences in the place where I was awake, they were very different from my awake experiences, which were very real. In other words, I was awake in two different spiritual realms or dimensions and both were very real because I could see, hear and feel the effects of the dimension that those around me could not see. I could hear the conversations and see the facsimiles of the people who were present in the dark reality. Even though all of the experiences didn't seem to be bad ones they were all effective in creating real pain in my body. The example of me being used as a tool to provide this entertainment to others. The use of my body and limbs, which projected something very beautiful and picturesque for others to see, in fact, it created a painful pulsation of electrodes to my body in some way.

When I think of these things and remember them very clearly, there is not a way for me to convince anyone of how real these incidences were to me. Another experience I had was being told that I was in a foreign country and that they were going to take me back to the United States so I could be with my family. The television stayed on all of the time and primarily on world news channels, so all I saw were commercials and news that were not in English. They were being presented in another language, and it was a language I had not heard before, so I couldn't even pinpoint the dialect. I remember the manikin people made me aware that they would be getting back to the US soon so I could be with my family. Surely now I know that some parts of what seemed very real were not real to this realm of life, but it was a true experience that I was going through.

Can you imagine waking up with tubes on both sides, not being able to speak, with machines beeping and monitors checking your blood pressure seems like every 15 minutes? Also, with the EKMO life support, I saw blood circulating outside of my body whenever I looked to the left. Having the discomfort of a piece of plastic stuck in your throat and a tube in your nose to help you breathe along with a ventilator. People constantly come in adjusting you in the bed, adjusting the bed itself and adjusting all of your machinery and striving not to cause you too much discomfort. Being delusional with labored breathing, consistent coughing spells that could last 5 to 10 minutes deep in your chest and causing soreness to your stomach muscles where it now even hurts to cough.

Okay, now let's step back into the reality you are familiar with for a moment and see what was happening on this side of my mind's experience. Remember, these dreams were happening daily whenever I was sleeping. Sometimes I wouldn't know if it was night or day, which was my inquiry regularly in order for me to keep up with the days. There was so much distortion in my thinking it all seemed very real. I refer to COVID as a spiritual disease and although there are many physical aspects to the disease, I think that having the greatest impact or effect is the spiritual part of the disease. How it makes you believe to such a real degree that the things you are going through are really happening. I just felt so out of control. This experience was the ultimate and I finally made up my mind I just could not go on in this manner. I was having an awake delusion that somehow, I had a file box of records attached to my IV running through my right arm or the juggler of the wrist if there was such a thing. I remember thinking this is never coming off. I am stuck with this thing for life, so much so to the point of giving up. That was my "This is IT," I couldn't bear another difficult or painful symptom.

Then there was the encounter of this nurse. We will call her Janice for the sake of names. She had an African or West Indian dialect very heavily. She had beautiful dark skin, but her character was dark, and I could feel that every time she came into the room. She was the epitome of hell as a nurse. She apparently was a head nurse of some sorts because those were the only nurses who were allowed to be in the room with the patients alone. Emory University Hospital is a teaching hospital, so if any of the interns were in the room, a head nurse would have to remain in the room at all times with them. Whenever she would come in the room, once she got me situated as far as movement and bed changing, she would always tell everyone she could handle everything herself from that point. She was evil, she would make gestures to me that were sexual in nature, such as talking about my beautiful caramel skin and my hair, and she would rub my arms or legs in a more seductive manner as opposed to a caring manner. I could feel the difference in her approach. It was sometimes like a Doctor Jekyll and Hyde approach. She would tie my hands down tightly so that I couldn't move them at all. I remember once she was in the room and I felt this snatch in my hair, and then she commented, "Oh wow, she cut your hair off," but no one else was in the room, and when I went to reach to see (which I could barely get my hand up that far), she slapped my hand down and said no be still and immediately tied my hands down.

This was the most alarming incident I had with her. This particular day she had in her hand what appeared to be a box cutter. I can't say for sure what it was, but that is what it looked like to me. She gave me my meds and she always worked from my right side, which was the opposite side from the room cameras. I often noticed that all of the other nurses worked from the left, which was on the side of the camera, and recorded what they did as they worked, but she always worked on the opposite side. This particular day after she got me situated in the bed and washed me off, she apparently cut the IV that was in my right arm or punctured the tubing in some way. I only know this because when shift change came, the nurses would go over all of what they did, handing the oncoming nurse instructions for care, etc. When they came to my right side and pulled the cover down, the bed was full of blood where I had been bleeding out of this tubing into the bed. I felt the wetness, but I didn't know what it was until they pulled the covers down. She acted so surprised, but I knew she was responsible, but I could not talk to tell anyone. Also, this is the same day that I got the cut on my face that is close to my right ear and I remember her saying, "Oh, she cut you and your ear is bleeding." There was no one else in the room but the gentleman who was checking my ventilator. He looked at her kind of suspiciously but did not question or respond; he quietly left the room. She wiped the cut by my ear while he was in the room to make it look as though she didn't know what had happened, but she was just dressing the wound. The nurses worked 4 days on shift and 3 days off shift. During those remainder of her days, I remember praying and asking God not to let me go to sleep.

Even though I was in a lot of pain when they would ask if I was in pain and did, I need meds; I would shake my head no. My blood pressure elevated to the point where they said, "We think you need a little something to take the edge off because your blood pressure indicates something is wrong. We need to get you calmed down. I still couldn't talk, so finally, when the shift changed on the third day, I gestured enough, and I know it was just God to get someone to get the night nurse to give me pencil and paper, and I wrote out in a scribble enough that she understood that this woman was hurting me. I don't know who she told or what she did, but I know it was God answering my prayer. She had already expressed to me how her parents were Pastors and she understood I was a woman of God and Pastor. She had also been told that I sang, so she was very comforting enough where I knew I had to try to get her to understand that this other nurse was hurting me. She assured me that she was going to get me moved off of that floor and get the problem resolved. I remember her telling me I had to get some rest because she had been told that I had not been resting or sleeping. I finally, after slowly writing down about Janice (the evil nurse), went to sleep.

The next morning when I awakened, I was in a different room, and she let me know I had been moved to another floor where only the nurses who had access to the isolation floor could come and this person did not have that access. I never saw her again for the remainder of the time I was in ICU.

This was my crossover point in ICU. A gentleman came in who had on scrubs very early in the morning. He said his morning introductions and stated his name. I don't remember what it was, but I do remember his kind nature. He gently rubbed my hand as if he knew my heart because I wanted to quit at this moment in the process. I didn't want to go on now chained literally to a file box that no one had the key too! No combination and no one actually knew why I had this file box attached to my wrist, almost like a burden to carry. This was as real as me talking to you right this moment while typing these pages.

The gentleman said, "Please, Please don't give up." It was like someone had whispered in his ear that I was a done deal. I had no more fights. I didn't want to go on in any shape, form, or fashion. COVID nineteen (19), Sederia zero (0). That was the score and I was at a loss. I had tears in my eyes, shaking my head from left to right "NO," stating with conviction that I couldn't fight anymore.

This gentleman, for the sake of conversation, we will call him Paul. He had a full beard and reddish hair and brows. He was a natural redhead, not hard to remember because my daughter tends to be fond of redheads. In his soft, kind voice, he just kept saying, *"Don't give up; we are going to figure out this mess."* Someway this attachment needed to come off and not without the possibility from the looks of things of disclosure of the box's contents. He said to me, *"Promise me you won't give up."* Paul had been so comforting that I made him a promise that I would hold on until the solution came by shaking my head yes. This was about 7 a.m. on a Friday morning after the experience with the deranged nurse. They had obliged me and moved me to another floor if you remember. It seems that I fell asleep after having this conversation with Paul.

I awakened to a beautiful nurse's assistant who stated that this was her job removing difficult IV positioning. Now I could get myself out of this pickle. She told me her name and I remember I had to repeat it several times. We will call her Emerald because of her beauty. The two people seemed as though they were real and kind (Paul and Emerald). She was supposed to be able to get this box with the lock on it, which was attached to my wrist disconnected from the IV, so it was a very tedious procedure. The place where the IV was located in my wrist was a very odd place, but I found out later it was placed there because of COVID. My veins would not tolerate an IV anywhere, so they had to use this vein in my hand and the juggler vein in my neck to attach what is called a pick line so that they could take blood regularly. My veins had also collapsed as did my lungs and the pick line kept an open IV to continuously get blood without sticking me over and over. Anyway, she was very quiet but kept assuring me that she was going to get the IV out of my hand and that would release me from having the box tied to me like I was a prisoner. I must have dozed off to sleep in the process because I remember her working on it diligently and having to take several different approaches. She finally got it off and loosened from the handcuff. I was so happy.

It seemed that everything that had been done inappropriately on the other floor they made corrections for on this isolated floor. They told me that I was on an isolated floor where this woman (Janet) could not come because you had to have special access to get on this particular floor. I never saw Janet again who had done these inappropriate gestures. I was glad, so I could finally get some sleep and not be afraid. The worst part of being in this position is not being able to speak and striving to get someone to understand your needs. Not being able to relay to people what you are going through. I remember how the panic set in because I knew that I was there alone and I couldn't speak or communicate with anyone. I couldn't even recall ever hearing if my family called or even if they knew how I was doing. The feeling of isolation when you are that ill is like nothing else you can imagine. The fear of not b knowing on both sides if they are properly trying to take care of you or not. Every time someone came into the room, they were changing me, moving me, or medicating me heavily. They would ask if you were in pain and sometimes, before I could say yes, they would proceed to go through the routine of giving me the medications.

I couldn't fight or argue, so basically, they did what they thought was best. I didn't have the fight to stop them from medicating me. I wasn't sure, without being able to talk, if it would be wise for me to go without medication because I was in so much pain most of the time that I remained in ICU. The pain medicine cocktail that I received was very strong. I heard the names of the medicines and most of them I was familiar with from other times I had been in emergency before I had back surgery; Dilaudid, Morphine, Benadryl, and Oxycodone were the main pain meds that I remember hearing them speak about. There may have been more, but when you are that ill to the point where they keep you comatose, you are really at the mercy of whoever is taking care of you, and all you can hope is that you are not being fondled or molested in any way. I was leery because of that one nurse that things could have happened to me, and I would never know, ever. This is a time when all you have is your faith and trust in God.

STAGE 3

As I began to stay awake more and more, the routine became familiar as to the timing of medications and what would happen day to day. As long as I was in ICU, which was 40 days exactly, I did not eat or drink anything by mouth. I had no water, not even ice chips, and after the experience with the crazy nurse (whom we will call Janet), now I was in really high anxiety. I also developed a temporary form of diabetes which meant they were constantly pricking my fingers to test my blood sugar. I was also getting insulin shots in my stomach and regular pricks to my fingers. Everything equaled pain, and to top it all off; I was sick.

Now comes the first stages of striving to bring my body to life, waking up my muscles. Although your mind tells you that you can do certain things as you try to do them, you learn that you cannot make your muscles and things work without using them. My body was like a vegetable. I couldn't do anything; every part of my body felt like a piece of lead when I tried to move it. I thought as I got well, my body would just automatically start working; that was not the case. I was experiencing as an adult what babies probably go through in their natural stages of development when they learn how to walk, talk, sit, stand, eat everything. I didn't even have control over my bowels and bladder initially, so even that was something that I had to develop mind control over again. We take these things for granted when we can easily do them day to day. When we have the luxury of doing it on our own but redeveloping these same attributes as an adult is very frustrating because you know that these are things you should be ableto do, but you cannot.

Thinking (because I am still at a stage where I can't talk yet), if I could just get out of the bed and stretch and get going with my life now that I am awake, I would probably feel better. Since no one can hear me, they don't know that I am ready to get going; boy, was I in for a rude awakening. The first time that I remember speaking to my kids, I got a chance to see them on facetime. It was such an overwhelming experience, I cried, but it was a joy. Then the depression came because although I spoke to them, I couldn't touch them, and they couldn't touch me, and I didn't know if I was going to make it out of there to ever see them again. Some moments I felt hopeful and like I could conquer this battle, and then there were bad days where I didn't even want to conquer the battle because it was so hard. It is like your body is fighting against you all of the way. The harder you try to get better or will yourself to better health, then your body begins to feel bad all over again. You aren't really sure if you are getting better or worse day to day and sometimes moment to moment.

Just as a reminder, the story may be random. I am writing as I remember because being inside the hospital with nothing but a clock, light, darkness outside, and sleeping for extended periods of time because of medication keeping a regular time clock in your mind is virtually impossible. As I was saying back to when they finally started to wake my body up, they had to start some sort of rehabilitation. This was done by lifting me up with what I refer to as a bed crane. They would strap you into this machine that literally looked like a crane so that they could lift you and all of your equipment safely. That was a process because some things could not be unhooked, like the ECMO, for example, or the ventilator, so just getting you in the crane was a task. Once the movement begins, that is when you realize how much pain you are in and how your body does not work any longer on its own. At this point, your body weight is working against you, not with you, and moving your toes can even seem like a process. My toes had been immobilized so long that they felt like they had rubber bands around each toe, tightly cutting off the circulation. I had no feeling whatsoever in my feet or toes. I remember I kept trying to see if there were rubber bands around each toe, wondering what would be the purpose of that, but I couldn't see my feet well, and I couldn't ask. The first time out of bed, I cried. It was so painful to my body and although they attempted to be as gentle as possible because you can't talk, you can't direct them as to what movements would be less painful. My experience may have been a little worse because I already had an injury to my back. This was not their greatest concern, nor did they take any consideration to the problem because I was not able to talk. I was not at a Kaiser facility where these records would have been a part of my file, so they would not know if this information was not disclosed. The way they moved me around or whatever they did when I was unconscious could have caused more damage to my back than anything else. This became another contending issue in my recovery to walk. Once I was in the crane, they moved me over to the side of the bed. The goal is to start out by getting you to be able to sit up on your own. They set you up, which feels good just because it is now a different position from what you have been in for weeks. It is also a painful position because every part of your body is a weight. My mind said I could move my legs and arms and do this and that, but the truth is you can't do anything your mind is telling you that youcan do. I was at that moment encapsulated with fear. Would I ever be able to walk or use my limbs the same way again? Had COVID intruded into my life, and I would not be that same person that weeks ago was walking, talking, driving, and being very independent only now to be a dependent vegetable of a person? Did they know enough about it to even guarantee that I would ever be the same? I had all of these questions and no answers because no one could hear the screaming in my head of fearful questions.

This was the beginning of the COVID-19 shutdown. They had not even figured out how to get people to survive this disease. A protocol of steps to definitely say this will save her life wasn't developed yet. I was the test that they would use to save other people, and I didn't even know it. All that meant to me is that they couldn't guarantee that I would be the same person. They didn't know, and all I could do was pray in my mind and hope for the best and believe God would work a miracle in my life and heal me in my entirety. It hurt so bad to be sitting up hanging in this crane; every part of my body was in pain. It's terrible when pain is how you gauge whether or not your body parts are dead or alive. **When pain gives you hope,** in this case, the pain was all over my body which was a good thing.

It was good because I had been so ill until I just didn't think I would make it. This pain, no matter how bad it was, gave me hope. I knew hanging there that I could feel in my body which meant I would be able to regain the use of my legs and arms. I wouldn't just be a vegetable of a person who has great thoughts and no way to move into action. Each day they were supposed to sit me up for 2 (two) hours at a time. There were times that they sat me up and I would be sitting up for some hours. It was torture because I couldn't cry out or rebel in any way. I wanted to let the nurses know how much pain I was in and I couldn't. I couldn't reach the pull cord to let the nurse know that it was too much and I was in pain. Sometimes I would hang there and cry. I remember this one incident especially, Nurse Janet was there, and she got me prepared to sit up. She knew I hadn't been able to do this on my own, so when she got me up this particular day, I remained in the crane for over four (4) hours just out of spite. I tried to bang on something, but nothing was within reach. She left me in that position for the remainder of her shift. The night nurse finally came in and removed me from the crane. Once again, I was in no position to complain or make it known how much this position was hurting me.

Obviously, I was getting stronger, I was staying awake longer, and finally, the day came when I was released to go to long-term care. It was very close to the end of May, so I had been in the ICU for approximately 40 days, and I knew this was a step in the direction to home. As much as I wanted to go home, the thought was frightening. What if I couldn't ever walk again? What if I would always have to be on oxygen? I was sent to an area where I was in isolation for a temporary period of time because they needed to wait to be sure that I was COVID-free. I didn't know what the test was like, but I had been poked and prodded so much I just didn't want to have anything painful happen, not even this test, but I was going to be in the isolation room until I took the test. I had developed fear of any kind of pain because I had been in so much pain previously and had been mistreated that the thought of them inflicting any kind of pain on me wasn't something I was willing to go through. I still had the tracheotomy in my throat, so I didn't want to have anymore tests.

STAGE 4

The room was very small; although it had a great view of the outside during the daytime, it would be extremely hot, and at night it would be freezing. I couldn't get the attention of the nurses by using the buzzer because they were always just too busy. I found out later it was because I wouldn't take the COVID test, so they only did what was absolutely necessary, and because the room was so extreme in temperature, the nurses wouldn't stay long, and the treatment was very different from ICU. In one incident, I woke up out of my sleep in a panic because it was so hot, I couldn't breathe. I tried to get the attention of the nurses. I pushed the nurse's button repeatedly and even used my remote to bang on the side railings hoping someone would come and finally, I began to pull at the ventilator so I could get it out so I could breathe. The nurse came in the room just in time as I was tugging on the ventilator trying to get it out because in my mind, it was the reason I couldn't breathe, and by now, I was taking short breaths feeling like I was going to pass out any moment.

Upon entering the room, the nurse was totally panicking because whatever tube was supposed to be connected to help with my breathing somehow had come unattached to the machine and it sounded the alarm at the nurse's station. God still was taking care of me because the isolation was really just that to the point that I could go 4 to 5 hours without no one coming to see if I was okay. When they would come, I would have to try to remember everything I needed, but my brain was still not a full capacity, so I would lose my thoughts quickly. I would have to repeat it over and over in my head to strive to remember to relay the information to whoever would come in the room. At this time, I was able to eat ice chips but still had not had solid foods. I finally committed to taking the COVID test after talking to my daughter and finding out what they were saying would hurt would only really be a feeling of pressure. I just knew I had to get out of that room after that incident; it was too hot, and I wasn't sure if they would be there to help me if something really went wrong because it seemed they were just ignoring me.

The following day I took the COVID test and still had to wait for three more days for the results. In the interim, the next order of business was to prepare me to remove whatever was impeding me from eating and drinking. I wanted so badly just to drink a full glass of water. Anyone who knows me knows that it had to be God because I never drank water if I could help it. I had this unending thirst for water and sunshine tangerine popsicles. They asked me what I wanted if I could eat. That's what I came up with, tangerine popsicles. I still had not regained my taste, and everything had a very funny smell, not foul but not good, but it was like my smell has heightened. I had no desire to eat much of anything just wanted to quench my thirst. During the three days that I waited for the test results, I was being taken through the process of taking me off the ventilator and removing the tracheotomy. I found out that removing the tracheotomy wasn't as easy as taking it out and then I could start eating. They had to test to see if the muscles in my throat were working properly, meaning that the windpipe closed properly when I swallowed. I never thought of myself as having muscles in my throat, in my neck, yes, but not in my throat. So, when the food came, it would go down the esophagus. They also had to make sure there wasn't scarring in my throat that would prevent me from talking again that the vocal cords were not damaged. All of this was very scary for me; my gifts and callings were in my throat, my teaching, singing, and counseling required me to use my vocal cords. I didn't care as much about eating as I did about talking and singing.

The day they removed the trach, I still had an open hole in my chest or throat, so they had to put this vocal box in the hole where the trach had been while the whole closed up. It was quite amazing because when they removed the oxygen and put the voice box in, I could talk. Each night they had to remove the voice box and place the oxygen back in because I could only keep the voice box in during the day and could not sleep with it, so at night, I couldn't talk. The COVID test came back negative, so now I could go into what they considered population with other patients. I was still in long-term care, but I wasn't in the small room anymore where everyone could ignore me. When they tested me for swallowing and eating again, they were amazed. They said that my muscles in my throat were intact; they didn't expect that result because I had the tracheotomy so long. I remember when I heard my voice after 47 days, I cried, and so did the nurse who took me through the process on how to slowly begin to eat and drink. I was only on clear liquids for 24 hours. Then I was onto solid food, which again, from my understanding from the nurses and doctor, was really impossible, more like unbelievable, another miracle. God was proving himself to me over and over in this miraculous recovery. I know that with every movement of progress, it was God. I was healing so fast that they couldn't even understand it except for the nurses and doctors who actually were believers.

Once I could talk, the behavior of the staff changed because now, I was able to advocate for myself what I did and didn't want to do or eat or drink. I had a voice, and trust me, I was using it because so many things; even though it may have been a part of saving my life, I could refuse because I could talk. Without your family being there, it is very scary because you can't advocate for yourself. I had come to the place in my mind and heart where I couldn't be humble enough. I had become aware of where I came from and the state of our nation with the pandemic. At that moment, I cried in sorrow but also in the joy of how much my God loved me out of millions of people. I woke up to civil unrest, police choking out people on TV, young folks being tazed in cars, and God speaking to me, letting me know this was a plague. Not something of the enemy but from the Creator of All of Things. I just wanted to know his purpose for saving my life, what was it that he wanted me to do. I knew something had definitely changed in my life. I was not the same person. Some of me or all of me died through this experience. The part of me that was suicidal, ungrateful, faithless, uncertain of God's Word being true because of the five years of storms and loss I had been experiencing prior to COVID. I asked God to give me understanding about my life, my purpose, and my continued destiny.

This place that you find yourself in when you go through something so close to death is a place of renewed strength and mind. Everything becomes about God and life and his people. Now after about 18 days in long-term care where I moved three different times in my room. I was in the room alone, and many nights it was difficult to go to sleep because I had the anxiety of someone coming into the room doing something to me. I still wouldn't be physically capable of running or fighting someone off. I think at times I would be sleep-deprived, and then I would sleep for long periods of time. Still having illicit dreams and high anxiety. Still having extremely bad heartburn to the point of feeling like I was having a heart attack. So many complications from being that sick in your body everything is rejuvenating itself. I learned what a baby feels like in this part of the experience. This is when I found out exactly what it feels like to be a little baby. The nurses would come in at 5:00 a.m. to bathe you and they would strip you naked and wash you down in the cold air-conditioned room. They move you from side to side to clean one side at a time. It was a good feeling once the whole process was done, but when you can't complain about how cold you are or ask them to cover you while they change the water and rinse the soap off, you lie there in the open freezing. One time I was shivering so severely that they finally asked me if I wanted to take my bath at night instead of mornings. Even the process for someone else brushing your teeth, it's all very strange when you had previously been able to do these what you considered simple tasks alone.

Recovery was not becoming as difficult as being ill. Either way, every part of the experience made me grateful and brought with it a greater humility than I had ever known. Finally, they began to work on my standing and going to the restroom on my own. So that initially created the task of me just getting on and off of the machine that they would use to take me back and forth to the potty chair. This was my daily chore to move from the bed to the toilet and from the toilet to a reclining chair on my own. Those five to ten steps may have been a mile because that was the degree of difficulty I felt. My body was heavy and my back was so sensitive to the point of anything I did in excess it would cause pain to my back or tailbone or both. No one seemed to be understanding of this point. They were now on the clock of insurance and what it would pay for in the rehabilitation process. I learned these things from the nurses; they would share certain things with me as they became attached to me. I remembered my Mom telling me when you are under the care of someone else. You don't want to make them angry because then you are at their mercy. Some of the nurses were just mean, and some had a servant's heart, but most of my caretakers, for the most part, were caring. I had that one nurse that I willnot forget the things she did to me and how she treated me.

   I got the speech about how I had to put forth a greater effort to regain the use of my limbs, but I just didn't have the strength at that point in the recovery. I wanted to in my mind, but it was not in my body yet. My back was really working against me, but again the concern was how much time would the insurance cover. Once you gain consciousness, it is a matter of the clock on your insurance. They began to put pressure on you to get to a point where you can walk with a walker, bathe yourself, take care of your general hygiene. Make sure you can make it up and down steps. You also played skill games to make sure your mind was intact, so I had to do puzzles, coloring, word games, and puzzles to test the cognitively of my brain. I found out at that point that I was going to have difficulty in my thinking and that made me sad. I also learned about my vanities and the areas in my life where I had pride. Thinking that I would not be able to use my mind in the same manner as before was a sad moment. I knew and believed that if God could bring me through everything I had gone through my mind was going to be a piece of cake. In my humankind, my pride was broken; I was bankrupt once again in my life. I had lost everything

everything and this time as before, I lost a greater part of who I thought I was because of this experience. I knew I was called to teach the Bible and that I loved to sing, and I loved doing church, as usual, being the habitual complacent church member but not really serving in spirit and in truth. I definitely had not come to the point before now to speak and teach the revelation that God had been giving me all alone about the dead bondage spirit in the churches. I am not saying that when I taught, I didn't teach the truth but not in the way that God had been showing me for years because of fear. After this type of experience, COVID 19, fear goes away.

Finally, after being told that they basically were not able to push me any further in the long-term care and because I could speak and rebut and do so many things without their help, I was told they were going to move me on to full rehabilitation. I was totally against it because I felt I needed more time for my body to get stronger, but the time had come to move on to the next phase. There I would begin a rigorous regiment daily to bodybuilding and muscle training doing everything with minimal assistance. Again, it was another grueling process because I had to go to a different facility, and I was struggling with anxiety and fear of what was next. They told me it could be as soon as the next day I believe that was day 17 in the long-term care, that they never thought I would survive to get through any of this because again, you have to realize they didn't know how to treat what I had. It was a test, and it looked like it was working, but even they knew it was a miracle that my recovery was so quick that they couldn't deny the power of God. We all know that doctors don't do that, but again, I was healing so quickly they just had to say this is our miracle.

STAGE 5

The very next day after breakfast, they came and told me that they were going to move me to the facility where they would get me prepared to go home. Although I was excited at the fact that no one would wake me up what seemed to be 100 times a day, I was still afraid that I wouldn't be able to manage on my own, and I still didn't know what to expect once I left the hospital. I had days where I felt absolutely sick, indescribably sick where there just were no words to tell anyone how bad I felt. I was moved the very next day. My physical therapist came to tell me that since I had gotten to the point where I was not taking instructions well from her, she thought it best that they fast-track me over to the rehabilitation area so that I could begin to prepare to go home. What she didn't understand is that I was not always feeling well enough to do some of the things they were striving to push me to do. Either way, I was taken by ambulance to another Emory facility for rehabilitation, and the hardest part of the physical rehabilitation began. Once they got me there, I was placed in an individual room with a television and a very modern hospital bed almost twice as wide as the older beds and fully remodeled rooms. The first day was quiet. I was left alone and told that my schedule would begin the next day. Enjoy the rest of my day of quiet because, after that, I would be on a constant schedule for recovery of the use of my legs and maneuvering to the restroom on my own, dressing myself (as my children had been asked to bring me clothes and shoes), bathe myself and take care of my own hygiene. I hadn't had my hair done or anything since I got there. It had grown quite a bit, but I knew I was going to need to redo it myself. I guess my illness still had not totally destroyed my vanity. You might think this would be the last thing on my mind, getting my hair done since I almost truly died but this too is another symptom of COVID. You have to overcome an enhanced feeling of insecurity. I was so depressed about so many different things, I felt as though I had done something to make God really angry for him to allow me to befall such a horrible disease. My mindset was so unsure of my relationship being in right standing with God. The things I saw or remembered in a comatose state were more real than the things I now experience from day to day. I also experienced extreme anxiety and a feeling of being afraid. Every emotion was so intensified, and I seemed to be confused on and off. It was hard to put my thoughts into words and I could not process how to speak about them or place them into the appropriate words.

Now the work begins, I had to find out if I could walk again and if I could get my lung capacity strong enough to keep me from having to go home with an oxygen tank, or at least that was my goal. I was given a schedule every day of therapy, along with constantly waking me and pricking me for diabetes and insulin shots in my stomach. Two (2) things were happening unexplained, I still was experiencing diabetic numbers in my blood sugar and I began to experience what felt like mild heart attacks. I remember this one early morning; I had eaten and then I really felt like I was having a severe heart attack. The nurse thought it was something muscle-related, so she ordered a cream and massaged my chest and back so that I could get comfortable going to sleep. I hadn't ever experienced pain that badly in my chest. I had all kinds of concerns because of having that tube in my chest (ECMO going through my heart). I thought perhaps I had really damaged my heart. I didn't realize that indigestion or acid reflux disease could cause symptoms closely related to a heart attack. Now I had to be placed on an additional medication after finding out that I had severe acid reflux disease, which I still suffer from today, almost a year later.

Every morning I would be awakened at approximately 5 a.m. to take my thyroid medicine and allow myself to go back to sleep until my first therapy class, whatever that might be. There were a series of classes such as speech therapy, physical therapy, cognitive therapy, and occupational therapy. Then I had the one class that allowed you to do what was considered fun therapy. It was like having a job and after being without a schedule and not having the strength to even lift my arms, now I have to do everything on my own. The therapist would give me a little assistance here and there. I had to have this belt that resembled a seat belt around me that was connected to the therapist so that if I lost my balance, they would be able to assist me quickly. I hated it because it reminded me of the thing that they put on babies when they are out shopping and they don't want to lose the child. It is this kinda harness like thing around them and me at the same time. Walking was the hardest of all of the things I had to learn again. My back was so out of whack from being in bed so long. The pain that I was experiencing was so pronounced that even with all of the medications I was taking for pain, it was not enough to keep me at a comfortable pain level. I don't know if I had given you the official list of meds; Morphine, Oxycodone, and Dilaudid were at the top of the list. I also had another pain med, but it wasn't one that came home with me. I had blood pressure medication, but I had to take one to keep my blood pressure from bottoming out. I had insulin twice a day and pricks 1/2 hour before every meal.

The discipline of not eating other than the three meals that they provided per day was not so hard because in ICU, I didn't eat solid food, so I had to build up my stamina for eating and walking. Those were the two hardest adjustments. I couldn't eat very much, but I was thirsty like a bottomless pit. I could not get enough water, and for those people who really know me, that was a part of my miracle truly. I never drank water and now I couldn't get enough of it. It had become like soda (which I loved prior to COVID). After about five days of rigorous exercising and crying, they took me through the process of bathing and trying to put on my own clothes. Everything was a tearful process, everything. It was so hard and painful and I had so very little energy that I just wanted to give up. As I stated earlier, there were so many times where I just wanted to quit. My age, the pain in my body, and the intense mood swings kept me in a depression. The highs and lows of crying and struggling to remember simple things like how to spell certain words, words that I clearly knew I could spell or pronounce, but I couldn't say them, or my thoughts would escape from me immediately. These were some of the things that were the most frustrating and fearful. I wondered every day would I ever get back to normal. Then there were what I like to refer to as my battle scars. Going into the hospital without these nasty keloids and now coming out with very visible scarring on my neck, face, chest, and near my vaginal area. The most frustrating part about that besides the fact that it was painful and agitating.

Each day was a trial in itself, and as I stated, I really wanted to give

up I just felt like I had been through enough and now I was stuck in the middle. Although God kept me alive and I was grateful, a part of me just thought maybe it would have been better if I had gone the other way, as they say, into the light even though I don't remember seeing a light. The Holy Spirit reminded me of some of the things I said in my communication with God prior to my illness. I realized I was very angry with God about the previous five years, from my Mom's death in 2015 to the very moment. I had asked God to allow me to be alone because I hadn't had a period in my life where I just lived alone from the time I was born until my husband left me in 2016. Fifty-seven (57) years of my life, there was someone there to share it with, and now at the most difficult and crucial period in my life, I was totally by myself. I also had asked God about healing because I was always suffering in my back. Now I had a broken heart. I had proclaimed to Him, how can I declare to others that You are a miraculous healer if You have never healed me in a way that no one else could. Well, He showed me and answered those prayers of mine or should I say angry complaints, and yet He still allowed me to beat incredible odds by keeping me alive and healing me in record. I was able to still walk, talk, think clearly, and make it off of the oxygen, etc. Okay, I am jumping ahead a little because I have been striving to keep this storyline in a way that you (my audience) can follow this COVID virus. Understand its seriousness and what a person who suffers a severe bout of COVID will have to go through in order to recover if they are blessed to make it
through.

After those five days of rigorous therapy, I was able to take my first.

bath in over two months. I had to take a sit-down shower and it was exhausting. I never knew just bathing your own body could be so taxing They let me know that they were preparing me to go home in the next 5 to 7 days maximum. The real deal is that my medical coverage wouldn't allow for me to stay longer if I had a different carrier. I may have been able to stay longer in rehabilitation. They felt because I was progressing so quickly and because I didn't live alone that the use of the bed had become a little more important than my feelings that more strengthening was needed. I think my greatest challenge was going to be stairs, going up and down, and getting in and out of the shower. Standing for long periods had not been mastered, and sitting for long periods of time (these were the areas I still struggled). The other part was just fear of being ready to be on my own. Well, the day was approaching, day 70. I remember it well because it was right after a weekend and it was one day before my 13th anniversary in Georgia. The Holy Spirit brought this to my attention, letting me know that everything about my life was new. I had a renewed spirit even though I didn't think so at the time. I felt defeated, frightened, and alone even though I knew my children would be in the house with me. It was not the same as the nurses and all of the assistance I received with the different apparatuses. I just knew I had to make it because Father God kept me alive for a greater purpose than I could explain.

STAGE 6

It's **June 30th, 2020;** I am as ready as I'll ever be, stunned, amazed, and frightened this new life of mine is about to begin. I didn't know if I would ever walk again on my own and I didn't know if I would always have to be on oxygen because even in my rehabilitation, I couldn't seem to keep oxygen levels above 80%. My number had to be 94 and higher. Those were my goals to walk without a walker and to lose my oxygen tank. The anticipation of my daughter picking me up seeing her and my son again in the flesh for the first time after 70 days was overwhelming. What a treat and yet I felt so sad about leaving the hospital. The doctor explained to me it's like getting married and going on a honeymoon where you have all of these immunities, and then the honeymoon ends; now it's back to real life and real-life situations. Also, I didn't know what I would be facing. I had been informed that my car had been repossessed and a few other money issues had arisen while I was in the hospital so it was back to real life. Just managing the idea of getting strong enough to do the things I used to do was a lot for me to think about without real-life experiences.

One of the issues I had other than oxygen and walking on my own is anxiety, blood thinners, keeping my blood pressure from dropping too low and keeping my sugar levels up because I was still dealing with a little diabetes. I had also developed an inflamed esophagus from being tube fed and probably given certain food even though, like baby food, that went against my acid reflux disease because whatever pre-existing problems I had in ICU that was not the major concern. I had things now that I never had to deal with before COVID. My body stabilization even after 70 days was still very much off. I came home with a shoebox full of medications that I had to take on a regular basis, so that was another goal to get rid of "the shoebox."

I remember that day and the anticipation of being around people feeling very fearful of I could catch this horrible disease again. I wouldn't be in a sterile clean environment, so there were certain precautions I had to take. I set up for someone to come and clean the house monthly so that it could be sterilized and really clean. I also set up to have food prepared fresh for me so that I could eat healthily and not go back to my usual diet that wasn't so healthy. I would have these meals brought to me six days a week, two (2) freshly prepared meals a day. I drank smoothie shakes, tons of water and fresh fruit, bananas, watermelon, and green grapes. Everything about my eating was different and most of it, if I could eat a whole meal, tasted like cardboard, so it made my appetite lessen. I had already lost 42 pounds (which I was happy because I wanted to lose weight), just not through sickness. Building my appetite would help me build up my strength, and I knew this, so I wanted to do everything that would keep me as healthy as possible.

I was so very happy to see my daughter. I began to cry. People talk about tears of joy and I thought I had really experienced that before, but not until this day when I saw my daughter's face. I was so grateful to God that He didn't let me die yet. I now had an opportunity to let go of all of my frustrations with my children, repent, and ask their forgiveness if I had not and to tell them how much I loved them. Sometimes in our day-to-day living, we forget how important the people we love are to us. I just knew I wasn't out of the woods yet with the diabetes and the blood pressure and oxygen so I could waste one moment on petty foolishness. Once we got to the house, I was so grateful even though I had lost my home that where we had moved to had no steps because I wasn't strong enough to hardly make the two small steps into the house where we had moved. Father God is so far ahead of where we are and really knows what we will need. I learned that in the small victories of just seeing this whole thing unfold right before my eyes that he had it all planned and what looked so very horrible was already working out for my good.

I came in and got situated in my room and then reality set in that I was going to have difficulty getting in and out of my bed and getting back and forth to the bathroom with my apparatuses. I didn't want to be a bother to my children, so I had to make myself work harder at getting to the place where I didn't need any help. The bedroom was set up so that I had a place for the oxygen generator and all of the small carry-around oxygen bottles for when I needed to go out. I had to be very time conscious because the small tanks were only good for 4 hours, so we had to think about any travel that would take place even though most of the time I only went to the doctor and back. This new lifestyle, even though temporary, was pretty hard to navigate but really only brought me more and more gratitude. I had to develop a routine that would work because my short-term memory had been affected severely. Even though I was cognitively aware of my surroundings and I could think the same, I could be in the middle of a sentence and completely lose my train of thought and couldn't retrieve it sometimes for days. I couldn't even remember to write down the thought so I wouldn't forget, and to this day, as I am writing about the experience 10 months later, I still suffer with that issue. It is not quite severe as it was but it is still there. I also fell into a deep depression with just the thought of maybe having to be dependent on my children for the rest of my life because I still didn't know if I was ever going to walk without a walker or breathe without an oxygen tank. I could feel the pain in my left lung whenever I would take a deep breath and still do today. I don't know if that will ever be normal, but I have to be grateful every day that I survive because I still know it is by miraculous design that I am here.

Every day was a challenge, I was still having lucid dreams and constant thirst like I could never get enough water which of course, forced me in and out of bed more frequently. I had a hospital be ordered and delivered because it was too hard to navigate in and out of my regular bed because of the height of it, and even though I had a step stool, it was still a big chore to get in and out of bed and in and out of the bathroom. I never thought just bathing myself would be such a chore and I didn't have the patience with myself so that would create so much frustration because my mind was moving at one pace and my ability and bodily functions at another. Keeping track of whether or not I had taken my medicines was my son's job and because he is a very routine person by nature of his Asperger's, he would be on the meds like clockwork. He also would prepare my morning meal and my afternoon and evening meals where the freshly prepared foods so I didn't have to worry about being hungry or eating. I had a small refrigerator in my bedroom as well, so my drinks and small fruit snacks were always available to me.

Some days my anxiety would be really high, especially when I had to be out in public amongst people. The fear of getting sick again was scary and seeing people everywhere with a mask on and hand sanitizer the whole world had changed in 70 days. Then the unthinkable happened; out of nowhere, my medical insurance was canceled. The company that supplied the bed and oxygen were the ones who made me aware that I had no more coverage because they needed a payment in order for me to keep getting my hospitalization apparatuses (bed, oxygen, and tanks, bedside restroom, shower chair, etc.). I didn't know what to do but to have to deal with this at this point and time in my life was overwhelming. Here I was in the middle of my COVID recovery plan, and now I had no insurance. All of my doctors followed up everything with Kaiser, and the idea of me having to find every doctor that I would need brought tears to my eyes (cardiology, pulmonary, respiratory therapist, and oncologist). I also was in the process of setting up my steroid shots for my back so that I could do more than just lay in the bed because my back had been so severely affected by my hospitalization and lack of movement.

In spite of everything I had been going through now, I had to deal with this one of the most important needs that I had at this time during the recovery. I had to utilize my old address and a mailing address to get the medical started again and, unfortunately, report that my new current address was a mistake. I used my business address that was "covered" in the support area of Kaiser in order to get the insurance started immediately. I felt pushed up against the wall and didn't know what else to do in order not to stop the flow of all of my care. This solution worked and I was able to get my medical services started back in 30 days; from Aug to October, I had no coverage, and then they started the services again. These things should not happen to a person after a major life-threatening disease. I learned later that it is called redlining and is done frequently when a person incurs a huge medical expense at the cost of a government expense. Medicare is a government expense even though it is given because of the 42 years I worked and put money into the system. This created a drive in me that people much like myself who have gone through this horrible experience in other places may have lost more than I did and may not even have insurance at all. Are these people left to die? Do they lose their insurance and don't know what to do to figure it out. No one should have to go through the worry about how they will continue treatment in the middle of their recovery.

STAGE 7

After all of this, I finally slowly began to feel better. I still had horrible dreams and difficulty breathing, especially since now I had to wear a mask everywhere I went. I still suffer from depression and anxiety from time to time. I had to be weaned off of the drugs that I was given while I was sick. I have been told that there will always be a level of scarring in my left lung, and although a small amount of fluid was discovered under my heart, they did not see a need for urgency to do anything about either one of these conditions. My heart was stated to be sound and my lung was stated to be stable. I do have to still use an inhaler from time to time. I have also had to have epidural shots in my spine because of the breakdown in the disc in my back from lying sedentary for so many days and having degenerative disc disease. One of the greatest challenges to my health has been my back and my lung. I am more than sure other than God's ability to miraculously heal and intervene in our wellbeing. I will struggle in these two (2) areas permanently. My singing voice was affected to some degree because of my breathing and I have a seemingly permanent raspy sound of my voice, which is nothing in comparison to my life being spared.

Where I am today, I am able to walk on my own, talk with cognitive speech and think at 100 percent. Initially, I had trouble remembering how to spell words that I was familiar with and I still lose my thoughts in the middle of conversations, but all these are minor effects compared to how much worse it could have been. God has taken this horrible experience and created a whole new life for me from my testimony. Today I am asked to give my testimony on radio shows across the nation and I have even appeared on some internet television networks. I have an upcoming television testimony reality show and I have two people who desire to write about my story in their magazines. I only say these things so that we can believe God's Word that he is a healer, that he will turn your negative experiences to work out for your good according to your calling for his purpose. He really never leaves you or forsakes you and the enemy cannot take your life unless God gives it over to him. "Love the Lord your God with all of your heart, mind, soul, and strength. Don't ever give up on God no matter how hard it seems because he doesn't ever give up on us."

I went through a horrible illness and experience in one sense of the pandemic, but I also was one of the first in Georgia to survive this horrible disease with the severity of symptoms that I had throughout my hospital stay. Ultimately, I was labeled the miracle by the doctors and nurses. When my pulmonologist first saw me after leaving the hospital, tears came to her eyes because she said she thought she would never see me again. Yet, I survived, not so that I could be great or somebody but because God wanted someone who would speak about his power and greatness to anybody who would hear my story. At this point, I am striving to use my non-profit organization to build an advocacy program for long-term care COVID survivors like myself. This advocacy group is entitled "Clean Slate." Our government is making a provision for the rebuilding of the economy based on the loss due to COVID but not specifically targeting the survivors of this disease. People who may have lost everything during their illness. People who would retain a million or more hospital bills. My bill was 1,8 million for the hospital stay and another 205,000.00 for medications and other costs. My medical insurance only covered a total of

600,000.00, the rest of the balance is still outstanding and a balance that I will never be able to pay in a lifetime.

I am seeking people who have a heart to serve and compassion for those who have lost everything they worked for while they were sick or hospitalized with this disease. Also, the families who had no intentions of losing the family members that they have in the manner in which they have lost them. All of these people need help. I would like for the advocacy program to create a package much like the one that I utilized to help to get me back on my feet. Eating a certain way taking vitamins and minerals while being weaned off of all of the pain medications and drugs that you have been given while in the hospital. Also, I desire to educate people on the horrors of this disease. We also would like to be able to have at least one family member in each family who is able to visit the family member daily if necessary, to strive to ensure that the person is not being mistreated in any way who can speak on behalf of the person who is comatose regarding any long-term illness pre-existing that the person may have had before hospitalization. I hope that people through this book can see the need for a program of this nature and strive to help me reach the right people to get help for these families who are victims of loss and people who are survivors and have lost.

Father God, You are the one and true Living God. I hope I have written this book about my healing journey in every way that will give honor to You. I hope I don't ever find myself again in a place of lack of gratitude for Your love for me. I pray that I remain as trustworthy to You as You have been to me. I lift up my brothers and sisters everywhere who doubt Your greatness and that Your Word is truth beyond our own forms of truth. I pray that You be exalted in every word of this book that some life, person, family, doubter, or someone even on the verge of giving up completely can find themselves in the words of this book. It is the truth that is true always. There is nothing made up but everything, as I remember it, to the best of my ability. I give You honor, praise, and glory for the rest of my remaining years, and I pray to remain humble and represent You in all Ido and say from now into eternity.

Pastor "Amazing Grace," your child Sederia.

ABOUT THE AUTHOR

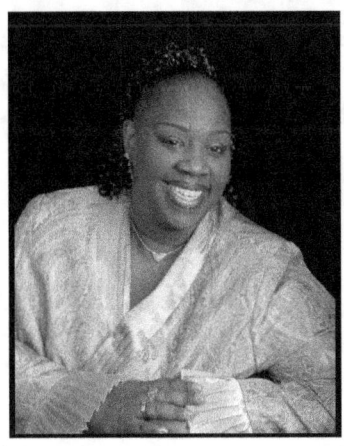

Sederia Graves was born in Cleveland, Ohio, but I spent most of my young adult to adult years in California. My writing was always a part of my life from as far back as I can remember. It began with poems mostly and a diary of things that would happen to me daily. As I grew older, I began to write about the things that I had difficulty sharing with others aloud as a release. I always had thoughts and ideas constantly flowing through my mind, but I could only write in confusion, tragedies, emotions, and things that we hard for me to touch basis within reality. I wrote poems and short stories, and as I developed my relationship with Christ, I began to receive revelation about His Word (the Bible) that I hadn't heard or studied before. I wanted to share the ideas and thoughts that I knew came directly from God, so I recently decided to write as many issues of these revelations as God would download into my spirit to enlighten the body of Christ. I hope they will help to bring clarity to some of your questions (as I had many) and refresh our thoughts and actions as a believer in the 21st Century. Enjoy and grow!

www.ingramcontent.com/pod-product-compliance
Lightning Source LLC
Chambersburg PA
CBHW071409070526
44578CB00002B/529